Thank You for HPV
A Simple Guide to Healing Yourself

Zeeluv Publishing House, Inc

Dania FL

Copyright © 2013 by Zayna De Gaia

Published and distributed in worldwide by:

Zeeluv Publishing House Inc, 2980 Griffin Road Unit5

Dania FL 33312

Book design by Zayna De Gaia

ISBN: 978-0-615-64983-2

Printed in the United State of America

This book is dedicated to the love of my life,
Moses Love

A NOTE FROM THE AUTHOR

This book shares my journey as a woman with HPV and how I overcame it. It's the same journey that many other women and men will encounter or have traveled. It is our journey, and one we walk together.

This book was written for you and anyone who has been diagnosed with HPV, Cervical Dysplasia, or Genital Plantar. It contains the steps you need to heal naturally and to stay healthy through diet, meditation, exercise, and a cleansing of the body and the mind. Because each component is so very important to our overall health, it is important that you read this book completely.

In the following chapters, I share with you my HPV experience from beginning to end. I openly expose the real and raw emotions, fears, and uncertainties behind my diagnosis and how I moved past them to effectively eliminate any trace of the HPV virus in my body. But most importantly, we will explore together how to have a healthy mind- which ultimately leads to a healthy body.

I know this works because it worked for me—it changed my life and my health. Now, I pass on the solution that will change yours.

As women, always remember that we are not victims of our bodies- but caregiver of our bodies. Therefore, the responsibility for our health and our healing should rest with the one person who has intimate knowledge of our physical, emotional, and mental health—our selves.

I invite you to read this book with an open mind and an open heart.

Let's begin our journey.

CONTENTS

1 WTF IS HPV ?

First off, I am not a doctor, neither am I giving any medical advice. I am sharing my experience, my opinions and my point of view. And what I am encouraging you to do is to do the same- do your research. Let this book be part of your learning journey.

I discovered I had HPV because I noticed I had warts. This may not be the case for everyone. HPV may not have any symptoms- which is why it's so important to get your recommended Pap screen and follow up with whatever your doctor tells you to ensure you don't have pre-cursors to cervical or other cancers.

It doesn't matter how this book got in your hands— what matters is how you use the information in it. You might need it for yourself, or maybe to help a friend or loved one. Regardless, this book will help to answer your questions and provide you with a resource toward your cure for HPV.

I wrote this book because I know how it feels to leave the gynecologist's office in tears after learning about an abnormal Pap test. I was scared and confused, and like you, I was full of questions about HPV but didn't know where to find the answers.

When I was 17 years old, I went for my yearly gynecologist appointment and was told I had something called HPV. After asking multiple questions, I left the clinic with no answers to this shocking news.

I walked out, like a zombie, opened the door to my car, sat in the drivers seat and sobbed my eyes out on the steering wheel. I was confused, upset, ashamed and I felt more alone than ever. I decided to ignore HPV and never talked about it to anyone again.

Years passed, Pap test after Pap test, my results turned up normal. A voice in the back of my head would say "They told you it could lay dormant forever… you still have HPV, they just can't detect it."

This shameful secret of mine made me feel like I was carrying some kind of weird "HPV Complex" – though invisible to everyone else, it tore at my heart and ripped at my self-esteem.

Fast forward 12 years later, I get my results back from my Pap test: ABNORMAL. They want me to come in again for further testing.

The news does not come as much as a shock- I've been waiting for the comeback- but I did not expect to feel so afraid.

I ask to see the head nurse, I have more questions about my abnormal Pap test.

"Mrs. De Gaia, you had some questions?"

"Yes, what do I do about this HPV thing? How do I get rid of it?"

"Well, since it is viral, there is nothing you can do about it Mrs. De Gaia. It's something you'll have, most likely, for the rest of your life."

"What do you mean for the rest of my life? What do you mean by "viral", can't viruses be treated?"

"Because it's a virus, it cannot be treated."

"So this surgery you are recommending- the freezing- it will only remove the symptoms, the warts- but we are not addressing the cause."

"This is what we highly recommend, at this stage."

"So what do you tell all the other women who come

through here and get the news they have HPV??"

"Well, you can work on boosting your immune system, that would help."

"How do I do that?"

"No smoking and no alcohol. Look up ways to increase your immune system."

"What about sex, can I still have sex with my boyfriend?"

"That's up to you. HPV is transmitted sexually. And can be transferred even when using a condom."

"So, I shouldn't have sex with my boyfriend? Well we've been having sex, so he probably has it to, right? How do I know if he has it?"

"Curently, there are no tests for men."

"hmmmph….."

"Any other questions?"

"How often do you have to tell a young woman that she has HPV?"

"Frequently. It's very common in young women."

"And there is no solution to it?"

"No."

This time when I walk out to my car, I am fully aware. I could smell the exhaust from other vehicles and I could hear everything around me. Unlike the first time I got this news, I now see this as an opportunity.

I open my car door, sit in the drivers seat and I put my hands on the steering wheel.

"Alright Zee. This is your test, your guru, your opportunity to heal yourself and to help many other women do the same. It's time to focus on YOU. Let's go to work."

I began my research. I studied, I investigated. I asked questions, I took classes and workshops. I empowered myself in every way I knew how – physically, mentally and spiritually. I took my healing very seriously- and I knew there was no going back. This was the beginning of a new chapter of my life. I couldn't wait to see the person I would become after this! I knew if I was going to beat this thing called HPV, it was up to me.

Thankfully, we live in the peak of the age of information. There is more information available to us than there has ever been in the history of humanity. It's both a blessing and a curse—a blessing if used wisely, a curse if not managed and not used wisely. My research uncovered some information that was refreshing, enlightening, and above all, relieving.

Today, I am HPV-FREE.

I'll never forget getting my Pap test results after I'd been doing all the healing work. I was nervous and excited. I called the automated message service and listened intently "The results of your Pap test", the automated voice said to me "PAUSE..... NORMAL"

Sigh.

"Wow.

Thank you. I did it."

I want you to be HPV-Free, too. If modern medicine does not have a cure for HPV, then you've got nothing to lose by choosing the natural method. It worked for me, and it can work for you.

And know this- every range of HPV, from mild to severe, can be reversed the natural way.

The journey of healing is a gift. HPV, or any other threat to our health, is a gift, wrapped in muck, but inside lies a brilliant gem—the gift of health and wellness that comes from knowing yourself and the motivation to create a new beginning in your life.

For most of us, an HPV diagnosis comes as a surprise. It's a shock and totally unexpected. Most likely you found out when the results of your annual Pap test came in with that dreaded phone call saying you need to go back to the doctor because the test results were abnormal. You were probably advised that abnormal cells were found, and while it's inconclusive what they are, they suspect it's HPV—Human Papillomavirus.

So nervous and anxious, you go back to the gynecologist for further testing, which confirms that, yes, you do indeed have HPV. You probably heard, in their scripted terms, that it's pretty serious and you should get treated. But then, they'll drop another bomb: they will treat you for HPV, but it's likely to come back in the future, and neither you nor your doctor has any control over that.

Well, that's great. You now have:

• An "incurable" sexually-transmitted "infection"

• An "incurable" sexually-transmitted infection that may lead to cervical cancer

• An "incurable" sexually-transmitted infection that, even when treated, may come back

• An "incurable" sexually-transmitted infection that may put you at risk of not being able to have children.

What the heck is HPV, anyway?

HPV is super common. It's actually epidemic. It is the most common viral STI and is likely to be the most common STI overall.

Many estimates have placed the lifetime likelihood of getting genital HPV to be in the shocking range of 75 to 90%. The risk of exposure to HPV is estimated to be approximately 15-25% per partner. And most people who get HPV never know they have it, as they do not develop genital warts, an abnormal pap test, or other manifestations of HPV that they can identify.

What about men? Men transmit HPV. This means that a woman has no way of knowing if her partner carries HPV because they are "silent" carriers. But, though the infection is usually invisible on men, they can and probably will transmit it to the next woman they sleep with.

HPV is a virus. It is transmitted sexually, and can lay dormant for years, undetected by Pap tests. Similar to the sprouting of a seed, viruses need fertile soil to grow. If placed on a counter top, the seed will not grow because it doesn't have the necessary ingredients. The seed needs fertile soil, water, and sun in order to grow and flourish. The same is true for a virus. A fertile ground for a virus to grow in is easy to create: throw in chemicals, stress, free radicals, and toxins like cigarettes and alcohol, and you have fertile ground for a virus like HPV to grow and manifest itself.

On the other hand, if you take the same virus and plant it in a clean body with a healthy, boosted immune system the virus cannot and will not grow.

It's simple. Clean up your body and your mind and you can wipe out HPV. It's a commitment and a lifestyle change; ultimately, it can be the key between illness and health

2 IT'S TIME
(TO CLEAN UP YOUR ACT)

W here to start?

Change your perspective, change your entire life.

But before we get in to the actual physical healing of warts, we're going to do a little cleaning. A kind of clearing of the space so we can go to work.

(By the way, yes, the warts can and will disappear. Though I am not opposed to any kind of surgery if you feel good about doing it.)

The first step to healing is to clean up your life. Look around you. Are you surrounded with what makes you happy?

Being committed to your happiness and striving as often as possible to be surrounded by things, peoples, and places that truly make you happy should be your number one priority.

I would say that to anyone undertaking any kind of healing from anything: divorce, cancer, HPV, or HIV. The #1 thing I would say to create healing is to focus on being HAPPY and feeling good.

If you are currently living in a toxic environment where you are unhappy, it may be time to make that change you know you've been needing to make. Being unhappy is a burden that will rob you of the potential to experience joy and pleasure that life has to offer. It also gets in the way of healing your body.

It's important to clean your environment of all negativity. Constantly watching the news, dramatic TV shows, and stressful movies can all have a harmful effect on our moods and also our bodies. Have you ever noticed what happens to your body when you watch a scary or suspenseful movie? You clench up, some parts of your body become tense, and your heart rate increases, beating hard against your chest.

We react to the things we watch, see, and hear. Our health is impacted every time we are upset. In order to have optimal health, contentment, and the best overall mental and emotional well being, we should try to avoid things that cause us stress, anxiety, or worry.

HPV breeds in a stressful environment. In fact, it loves stress, because stress is to HPV what oxygen is to you—LIFE!

Increase your intake of funny movies and TV shows, stand-up comedy routines, and any other uplifting activities that make you laugh and smile.

My personal favorite pastime is laughing yoga, basically laughing for no reason. Usually laughter is produced by using the analytical part of the brain, the right side. When you laugh for no reason, the left side of the brain is active which makes laughing even more healing. And it's a lot of fun.

Smiling and laughing are both amazingly contagious and make your entire body feel good. Look for reasons to smile, and opportunities to laugh often.

Exercise:

What brings you true joy?

What really makes you happy?

What makes you smile?

What makes you feel like a little kid all over again? Who are the people in your life with whom you laugh?

Ask yourself these questions and make a list of those things that make you especially happy. Then spend some time each day doing those things that bring you joy and make you smile (or laugh).

Here are some ideas you might include in your list (this is part of my personal list) :

- Taking a hot bath
- Getting a massage
- Having a girls night in or out
- Dancing/Singing

3 WHAT'S YOUR STORY?

Healing happens first at the soul level, which is above the mind and the body. As we heal the deep trenches of the soul, we heal the mind and we heal the body.

We see this often in our lives. Stress, grief, anger, or anxiety can all impact our overall health, causing stomach problems, headaches, high blood pressure, fatigue, etc. The natural way to cure those health problems is to relieve ourselves of the emotional or mental issues which are behind them—when they are gone, the physical healing will follow.

Finding out you have a sexually transmitted infection can be challenging emotionally. I know. On top of having HPV, I discovered that I carried a lot of guilt associated with contracting

HPV- and that guilt added to the loneliness and the fear.

Here's where my personal emotional healing happened. I realized that having sex and getting a virus does not make me any less of a person. I did not do anything "wrong". I got a virus. It came from a sexual experience that I consented to. That's what happened.

What my mind made up about the situation is a whole different story! My mind made up all these negative labels. And the deeper I dug, the more hurtful and self shaming the labels were.

Two different stories aren't they? The first one, is what happened. I had sex, got a virus. Period. I could have gotten a virus from someone coughing or sneezing. But I happened to get a virus that was transmitted sexually, not airborne.

The second story is made up from my mind, based on my past experiences and my perception of myself and the world.

Whatever story you've made up about yourself and your HPV- it's important to "see" it first so you can clear your mind of those stories.

Our mind works like a machine. Something happens, and our mind makes up a story about it. We believe the story. Then we live our life according to that story. And this keeps repeating over and over again.

Eventually, we're caught up in a bunch of stories that don't really apply to us and don't serve any good purpose, except to validate the mind's stories.

While we're so busy believing our stories, we forget that they're made up. There is no truth to them, yet we live our lives according to these made-up stories. It's critical to realize that our stories are completely made up by our minds and shaped by the experiences we've had in our life.

The story that came up for me was " I fucked up."—and all the stories that were created from there. I was all about taking responsibility for my life- but I had taken a wrong turn- I was blaming myself and making myself wrong.

I believed that I was at fault for every bad thing that happened and I convinced myself that the stories were true. Then, I simply kept repeating those stories to give my mind an opportunity to prove that the stories are right. (That's what the mind loves- to find proof to the stories).

In reality, what is real is not that "I fucked up" or

whatever else that my minds makes up— it's that I have a strand called HPV in my body. PERIOD. End of story.

Everything else is bullshit. It is what it is, a virus, nothing more.

And as for the other stuff, to be human is to sometimes make mistakes, and to grow, we sometimes find ourselves in relationships that cause pain that we can learn from.

It's all just the stuff of life-neither good nor bad.

Exercise:

Did you place blame on yourself, engage in self-criticism, or insult yourself because you found out that you have a virus? Did you beat yourself up?

Journal the answers to these questions:

1. You are diagnosed with HPV. When you found out, what thoughts rushed into your mind?

2. What story did you make up about YOU because you "got" HPV?

3. What does the fact that you "got" HPV mean about you?

"I was diagnosed with HPV; therefore it means that I am..." Complete the sentence and see where it takes you. Allow yourself to be really honest about it. The more truthful you are to yourself now, the smoother your healing journey will be. Remember, you can't heal or fix something that you ignore.

4 REWRITE YOUR STORY
(BECAUSE YOU CAN)

Please read this very attentively:

You are perfect exactly as you are.

You are perfect exactly where you are in your life right now—HPV and all.

As you know, life is a ride; it has its up and its downs. Roll with it, babe! Who you choose to be in the face of the challenging parts of your life is really what determines the quality of the life you will live.

In the last chapter, we discussed the stories that we create when life happens. Becoming aware that we do this is the first step to empowering yourself. Once you shed light on a story, it no longer holds the same power over you!

Byron Katie, one of my favorite speakers and

teachers in the world, created *The Work,* a method that teaches us to question disempowering or stressful thoughts or stories.

She teaches that a thought is harmless unless we believe it. It is not our thoughts, but the attachment to our thoughts, that causes suffering. Attaching to a thought means believing that it's true, without inquiring or questioning its merit or validity. A belief is a thought that we've been attached to, often for years. By questioning our stories, we begin to train our brain to see two sides of each story. This is how *The Work* works: it helps us to free ourselves from our mind.

Let's go to work. First, let's identify the stressful thought:

"I have HPV and it's a bad thing."

When "bad" things happen, our first thought is that things shouldn't be this way. That this is WRONG! It's unfair, it's not good, it's a misfortune, a bad thing.

So let's question this story, shall we?

Question 1: Can you be certain this is truth: "I have HPV and it's a bad thing"

Answer this question honestly. Are you sure that you having HPV is really bad? For real? You know this for sure? If you are feeling this is true, then the answer would be yes, it's true; I should not have HPV. Be still. If you really want to know the truth, the honest yes or no from within will rise to meet the question as you recall that same situation in your mind's eye. Let the mind ask the question, and wait for the answer that surfaces. Yes or no.

Question 2: Can you be absolutely certain that you having HPV is a bad thing?

Ask yourself again, this time, with more intention. Are you totally, absolutely sure, this is true? If the answer is still yes, that's perfect.

Question 3: How do you react when you have the thought "I have HPV and it's a bad thing"?

How do you feel inside your body when you think the thought? Be still, notice. Close your eyes and repeat your story to yourself. Get in your feeling body and outside of the thinking. Scan your inners for the sensations. Witness how you treat yourself in this situation and how that feels. "I shut down. I isolate myself, I feel sick, I feel angry, I eat compulsively, and for days, I watch television without really watching. I feel depressed, separate, resentful, lonely." Notice all the effects that come from believing the thought.

Contemplate the thought and really feel how you feel in your body when you think it. Sit with the feelings or the sensations it brings up. Does the area around your chest tighten? Do you feel icky? Do your shoulders tense? Do you get the jitters or butterflies in the pit of your belly? What exactly do you feel inside?

Our physical reactions are totally habitual. We get used to feeling them, and we forget that they are linked up with these stories, these thoughts, that we make up.

Question 4: Who would you be if you didn't have this thought?

Now consider who you would be, in that same situation, without the thought "I have HPV and it's a bad thing". Who would you be, what would you be like, if you did not have this thought? What if this thought, "I have HPV and it's a bad thing" did not pass through your mind? How would you be? How would you act?

Close your eyes and imagine sitting in the doctor's office learning you have HPV. Imagine yourself without the thought "I have HPV and it's a really bad thing" Take your time. Notice whatever is revealed to you. What do you see now? Notice the difference.

Without this thought, you'd be... happy? Perhaps free? Maybe just living your life, normally, being yourself. Going out with your friends. Going on with your life as usual!

The Turnaround

Next, you turn it around. The story "I have HPV and it's a really bad thing" becomes "I have HPV and it's a good thing"

You flip it.

Is that turnaround just as true or even more so? Now identify examples of how "I have HPV and it's a good thing" can be true. Find at least three specific, genuine examples of how this turnaround is true.

For me, one example is: I have HPV and it's a good thing, because the virus entered my body at some point and it makes total sense that I have what they call HPV".

Another example is: I have HPV and it's a good thing because I needed it to show me my ability to heal myself.

And one more is: I have HPV and it's a good thing because it has given me an opportunity to step up my game as the CEO of my life and really take care of my body and my mind at a high level.

This entire process is a meditation. You should take your time and meditate with each question and answer. Allow yourself to feel the process.

5 PRAYER AND AFFIRMATIONS

It's important to be in a positive state of mind, especially while you are healing. Prayer, meditation, repeating affirmations or mantras, and using visualization are all powerful tools to assist your healing journey.

When I first found out I had HPV and made the choice I was going to heal myself, I woke up before sunrise and headed to the beach. Being awake to witness the sunrise hour is very beautiful and peaceful—this is a very powerful time of the day.

I created a prayer/mantra that I still chant today.

"I am happy, I am healthy,
I am holy, I am healed.
Thank You God, Thank You God,
Thank You God, Thank You God."

I sing these affirmations to myself for 10 minutes, as a form of prayer, feeling each one deep in my cells. Since what we focus on expands, it is important to verbalize what we are creating and let the Universe know what we are focusing on.

Many cultures will affirm that this early morning time is auspicious, a time to be in communion with God, the universe, whatever you want to call It. Repeating a positive mantra first thing in the morning sets your mind for the rest of the day. Why morning? When you wake up, the mind is in its purest form—it is as clear as it will be for the day. It is refreshed and receptive to everything. Once you get started with your day, though, the mind becomes cluttered with outside influences, like work, conversations, news, responsibilities, worries, etc.

It's important that affirmations like these are spoken with belief. Simply reiterating them, without believing them deep inside, will not produce results that are as effective. Affirmations are a way to infuse yourself with positivity, a powerful healing component. So in order for that positivity to work wonders, we must develop faith that it will. Our body will then accept it more readily.

One of the most powerful mantras I know comes from the Hawaiian healing technique Ho'oponopono. It's simple and it works.

"I love you

I'm sorry

Forgive me

Thank you"

Repeating this mantra to yourself will create healing and miracles in your life. If you don't have a mantra or positive affirmation for yourself- this is a great one to adopt right away!

6 GRATITUDE

Gratitude is an important ingredient in the healing process. I called this book "Thank You for HPV" to get your attention and also because your attitude towards this thing called HPV is super-important.

It is totally normal to feel upset, sad, and angry about having HPV in your body. If you need to cry, cry girl! If you need to scream, do it! Get it out so it does not stay stuck in your body- and then take a deep, deep breath.

Gratitude is a special gift that gives us access to our manifestation powers. When we are grateful for what we have, and really take the time to feel deep appreciation in our hearts, we enter a state of bliss. Gratitude is a gateway to heaven on earth. It has a powerful effect on our mental, emotional, spiritual, and yes, even physical well-being.

When you first wake up in the morning, it's an opportunity to count your blessings and thank God for another day. None of us are guaranteed another day, or even another breath. Every time we wake up to a new day, it's a gift, another go at being human on this planet.

It's a special gift to have access to gratitude for everything—both the good and the bad. That gratitude gives us a different perspective, and it empowers us in our daily life.

Being able to genuinely express gratitude requires you to *shift your focus* away from the things that are negative and toward those things for which you feel thankful for. And as you already know, it's very easy to forget to be thankful for all the amazing things we experience on a daily basis.

Here's a list of some of the things for which you may find plenty of gratitude:

•Your health. Even if it isn't perfect, you may be thankful for the health you have. Regardless of what state it is in, without health, there is no life.

•Your family.

•Your freedoms

•Your intelligence, consciousness, and awareness.

•Your memories!

•Sunshine and nature

•Food and seeds, some of the many remarkable gifts from Mother Nature. It's nature's natural way of sustaining us.

•Your job, business, or career which provides the income you need.

•Your pets/animal companions.

Here's the deal: you can be grateful to have an illness or injury. That's the key. I know it sounds a little crazy being grateful or appreciating a virus in our body. It is this perspective which gives you access to healing.

For example, if you've been diagnosed with HPV, you might consider being grateful for:

•HPV in my body, because it allows me to grow and know myself as a healer.

•HPV, because it magnifies my life and has inspired me to choose a new healthy lifestyle. Thank you for HPV and the opportunity it gives me to make my body better, stronger, and healthier.

•I am grateful for this healing journey, because it is giving me the strength to take on a new lifestyle and shows me that I am a healer.

•I am grateful for the challenges in my life for they make me appreciate the good things in my life even more.

•I am grateful for the infection in my body for it makes me stronger and makes me more committed than I have ever known myself to be.

I know former "cancer patients" who are convinced that "cancer is the best thing that ever happened to them" because it helped set them on a new and better path than they had been on before their cancer journey. It helped them appreciate and take control of their life and their body.

There is a very *real healing effect* that is initiated in your body when you express gratitude toward people or things outside of yourself. Some of this effect can be measured biochemically, while other aspects of it are currently beyond scientific measurement. But the bottom line is irrefutable: Expressing gratitude initiates a powerful healing effect in your own mind and body.

Gratitude is the opposite of anger. You can be angry that you have HPV, but anger will be counter-productive to healing. Many people are angry, a great deal of the time. Some people express their anger, fully and regularly, and others hold it in and suffocate it. This can be really damaging to the body and can cause many kinds of problems. Remember, illness manifests at all the different layers of self— physical, emotional, and mental. Anger is a very destructive emotion because it causes stress, adrenal depletion and tension throughout the body. But you can learn to replace anger (or other negative emotion) with gratitude, and anger cannot coexist with gratitude.

In this way, gratitude begins to nudge out the other negative emotions you might be experiencing. This doesn't mean you have to run around, blindly thankful for everything, without discerning those times when criticism or anger might be called for—releasing and expressing our emotions is one way of detoxing them from our body and mind. However, the more you can *find gratitude in everyday things,* the more you'll activate and support your body's inner healing processes.

Hence the expression, too blessed to be stressed. Yea baby.

Exercise:

Every morning, write down 10 things you are grateful for. Then take a few minutes to contemplate your list. Bring your attention to your heart, and feel the deep appreciation you have for your life and those things you are grateful for.

7 MEDITATION
(IT'S A PRACTICE)

Meditation is a very powerful practice. It is known and proven that meditation alone can help to improve both physical and emotional health. A little a day, done consistently goes a long, long way.

First thing when you wake up is the best time to meditate because your mind is still fresh, not yet filled with the daily, "blah blah blahs." There are different forms of meditation you can practice, I recommend trying them all and finding the one you resonate with the most at this time in your life. You can change it up, too; you may prefer one method one day and another method on another day. It's all good as long as you are doing your practice.

Here, I'll introduce to you three different meditation methods that I use.

1. Kundalini Yoga and Meditation

Kundalini yoga is a powerful, powerful tool. I can share so many things that exhilarate me, but Kundalini is one that far surpasses any other forms of elevation I can do. I do it daily—it's a regular and consistent part of my personal regimen of happiness!

My favorite yoga book is called *I am Woman* by Yogi Bhajan. This book has many different exercises and meditations specifically designed for women to empower themselves. One of my favorites is the Self-Love Meditation. I recommend doing it for 11 days, 11 minutes a day – and see for yourself what will transpire.

Creating Self-Love, a Kundalini Yoga Meditation from the *I am Woman* book:

1. Begin in seated position. Hold the right palm 6-9 inches above the top of your head. The right palm faces down, blessing you. The left elbow is bent and the left palm faces forward, blessing the world. Breathe long and slow. Do your best to only breathe one breath per minute in this way: inhale for 20 seconds, hold 20 seconds, exhale 20 seconds. Repeat for 11 minutes. Inhale deeply and move directly and slowly into the second exercise.

2. Extend the arms out in front of you so the arms are parallel to the floor and your palms are facing forward. Long deep breathing for 3 minutes.

3. Extend your arms overhead with the palms facing forward. Long deep breathing for 3 minutes.

2. Breathing Meditation

Using your breath as the focal point of your meditation makes meditation accessible anywhere, anyhow. All you need is your breath, and I'm guessing you have access to that anytime, anywhere!

When we focus on our breath, our mind slows down, it zooms in a little more and it allows our entire nervous system to relax. This is important for day-to-day functioning and especially important when we are on a healing protocol.

This focusing of the mind on the breath relaxes the never-ending dialogue of the mind.

We all have a little voice in our heads that is commenting, agreeing, disagreeing constantly from the minute we wake up to the moment we fall asleep. This little voice is not the most positive voice- and it isn't that friendly either!

Meditation helps to observe that little voice and all the thoughts flowing through our mind and when we begin simply observing and not reacting to these thoughts, we can gain control of our life.

Clearly, we have no control over the circumstances in our life. Storms, hurricanes, earthquakes- they happen. What we do have control over is *how* we deal with these circumstances and that's what has the biggest impact on the quality of our lives.

Set a timer for your meditation. You can start with 5 minutes and work your way up to 20 minutes, and eventually 30 minutes a day.

One-minute breath meditation

1. Sit upright in a comfortable seated position and close your eyes. Begin observing your breath.

2. Inhale for a count of 5.

3. Hold the breath in for a count of 5.

4. Exhale for a count of 5.

You can keep increasing your counts: inhale for 6, hold for 6 and exhale for 6- eventually the advanced practice is inhale 20, hold 20 and exhale for 20 (hence the name 1-minute breath)

Repeat the 3-part breath until your timer goes off.

Sit for a few breaths before getting up, feeling gratitude in your heart for your life and for each breath that you take.

3. Nature Meditation

Being in nature is so soothing and relaxing. Anyone who's experienced the sweet sound of waterfalls or the relaxing effect of the ripples in a lake or the sounds of birds chirping can attest to the relaxing effect that nature can have on our human bodies.

I love to go out in nature- anywhere there is grass, a tree, water, sky, - and simply sit and observe. You can use different focal points. I love to sit and feel the wind on my skin. Sometimes it's very subtle and meditating on the subtleness is a great meditation. Or if you have the privilege of being by the ocean, simply watching the waves roll into the shore has a hypnotizing and relaxing effect.

All these meditations are effective and can create miracles in your life. But here's the thing- they only work if you do them. And no one else can do this for you, it's gotta be you, babe!

8 PHYSICAL EXERCISE
(GET OFF YOUR BUTT)

Exercising is essential to all human beings. Working out our heart muscles, strengthening and lengthening our muscle groups and stretching our body parts are all essential.

You must find the exercises that you enjoy. There is only one way to find out: TRY DIFFERENT ONES- till you find your workout of choice and roll with it. Roll with it, regularly and consistently.

Here are some of my favorite exercises. I love doing all of these activities and feel absolutely amazing in my body whenever I am engaging in them.

Yoga:

Yoga comes in all shapes and sizes. There are more kinds of yoga than brands of cereal! Try them all and find one that is right for you. You will feel amazing in your body and you will also think more clearly, be more patient and enjoy your life more.

If going to yoga studio is a little scary to you-start at home, that's how I started. I bought DVDs and I practiced in my living room

Dancing:

Dancing feeds my soul. If that's you too, than make it your workout! Belly dancing, zumba, hip hop – dance your butt off! Wear cute outfits, do your hair, shake your hips, do the shimmy!

Walking:

Walking every day for at least 30 minutes at a brisk pace keeps you vital and healthy. I like to walk in silence and in nature.

Exercise:

Make a list of your favorite physical activities and do some research online for places you can practice these in a group setting. For example if you like to dance, look for dancing classes. Want to try kickboxing or yoga? Look for local place that offers classes and sign up!

9 YOUR IMMUNE SYSTEM (BOOST IT!)

HPV is a viral infection, so the answer to booting the virus out is to boost your immune system. Your immune system is like an army of soldiers who are ready and willing to fight for you and protect your body. However, if your little soldiers are not fed properly, they will not be able to do their jobs. They'll become too weak and sluggish for the task at hand.

Phytochemicals are the main foods that nurture the immune system's army. Fruits, vegetables, tonic herbs and medicinal mushrooms contain phytochemicals that unlock our body's immune system, but most people don't get enough of them.

Phytochemicals often hide in the cellulose fibers of seeds, skins, stems and rinds of the fruits, and vegetables we eat. Many eat the right foods, but throw away the parts with all the medicine! For instance, they eat potatoes and carrots, but peel away the skin, which contains the richest nutrients.

Incorporating these critical phytochemicals is why smoothies made with a 3-horsepower blender are an important part of this healing protocol. There are 2 companies that offer these types of blenders: Blendtec and Vitamix.

We must break out or "micronize" phytochemicals from seeds, stems, skins, and rinds. A smoothie made with a blender that keeps the healthiest parts of fruits and veggies is so important. Some might think that using a juicer is sufficient, but juicing fruits and vegetables is a waste of time. It throws the fiber away, which is where phytochemicals dwell!

In the back matter of this book, I share my favorite healing smoothie recipe. One smoothie every day, preferably in the morning, is recommended. I generally have tea in the morning to help my bowel movement, then I do my yoga practice, and then I make my daily smoothie. I cannot emphasize enough the importance of the 3-horsepower blender and healing smoothies to facilitate healing. The blender runs about $400. Yes, it's a little pricey, but you are worth the investment. Consider the cost savings over hospital bills. All you have to cough up is a blender, which, believe me, will pay for itself time and again throughout the years.

Herbs to strengthen the Immune System

There are a multitude of natural herbs, mushrooms and roots that can be used to boost the immune system. Here are 3 that I recommend:

Astralagus is an herb traditionally used in Chinese medicine to regulate and maintain the immune system. Its anti-viral and anti-aging qualities are very important for healing a viral infection!

Agaricus, known as "God's mushroom" is widely used for to overcome numerous diseases relating to the immune system amongst other disorders. This is an immune system booster.

Reishi Mushroom, another magical mushroom revered in Chinese medicine, is used to reverse cancer, HIV, heart disease and much more. I recommend Reishi in everyone's diet.

What Weakens the Immune System?

• **Refined Sugar** – Refined sugar is an immune system suppressant! It hinders or destroys the immune system's ability to protect a person from germs, viruses, bacteria, cancer, etc. Every time a person drinks a soda or eats candy, donuts, cake, pie, pastry or anything else containing refined sugar, they are disabling their immune system, making it less protective. You cannot consume refined sugar and strengthen your immune system. Sugar must go. Even "Organic" sugar, must go.

I use Raw Agave Nectar mostly as an alternative to sugar. Personally I think the verdict is still out on Agave- but I believe it's better than processed white sugar. I also like to sweeten my smoothies and deserts with dates.

Stevia and coconut sugar are also good, healthy alternatives to sugar, but should be taken in moderation like any other sugars.

• **Standard American Diet (SAD)** – Our body's cells are dependent on the nutrients made available from the foods we eat. The SAD does not provide those cells with quality building materials, in fact it provides the opposite. Processed food, fried foods and salty canned goods are a hindrance to our health.

• **Cow's Milk** is responsible for most of the congestion and allergy problems people experience – this is true for children and adults. Cow's milk, organic or not, is a dangerous substance to place into the body of any human. God designed cow milk to nourish a 100-pound calf at birth and grow it to 2,000 or more pounds at maturity. He did not design cow's milk for human consumption.

• **Vaccinations** – The number of immune-destroying substances found in vaccinations is staggering. They contain detergents, formaldehyde, microbes, antibiotics, chemicals, heavy metals and animal byproducts, just for starters. We need to realize that when we allow these toxic substances to be injected into our bodies, we are doing great harm to the immune system.

• **Dehydration** – Most people do not drink enough purified water. Drinking liquids such as coffee, caffeinated teas, sodas, energy drinks, and alcohol, rather than providing the body with hydrating liquid, only causes further dehydration.

Other Immune System Killers

• Obesity and carrying excess weight

- Smoking

- Drinking alcohol and the use of other drugs

- Drinking chlorinated and fluoridated water

- Dying of hair (the toxic dyes are absorbed into the blood stream)

- Consuming artificial sweeteners and foods containing MSG

- Eating French fries and other fried foods.

- Watching television for extended periods of time

- Sitting in front of a computer for long periods

In short, the human body becomes susceptible to illness (like HPV) when the immune system is compromised. Unfortunately, modern-day diets weaken our immune systems and our body's army against illness and disease simply don't have what it takes to combat them. And we further impair the immune system's ability to protect us through our daily activities—we sit for long periods of time in front of TVs and computers, we don't get enough fresh air, sunshine, or exercise, and we choose social activities, like drinking and/or smoking, that disable our immune system. When that happens, we not only open the door to illness, but we give it full reign to overtake our immune system, zapping it of any ability to protect us now and in the future.

Exercise:

What are the activities in your daily life that are impairing your immune system? What healthier, immune boosting practices can you replace these with?

10 FOOD HEALING

It's time to take the next step in your healing journey- detoxing your physical body.

If you are serious about being healed, completely healed, it's important that you treat your body like a temple and eliminate any toxins that have taken up residence from smoking, drinking, eating processed food, and contact with pesticides. We will be focusing on super-boosting your immune system to serve your healing.

As part of your healing journey, it's important that you completely eliminate toxins such as cigarettes and alcohol. The fact is your body needs to be 100% optimal to heal, and smoking and drinking alcohol are toxic and dangerous— and they totally mess up your immune system.

Cigarettes

A short word on cigarettes- at one time,

cigarettes were not considered dangerous—people who were sick and hospitalized were even allowed to smoke! Today, however, smoking is a known violent act toward our body. I mean seriously if you're still smoking cigarettes- it's time to give them up.

Smoking can be harmful to the lungs, but that's just a small part of the health dangers posed by cigarettes. Smoking commercially created cigarettes is like putting yourself in a disgusting chamber full of chemicals. No thank you!

Oh, also if you smoke "organic" or light cigarettes, they are still a no-no. Anything that impairs the liver is out.

Alcohol

While you're on your healing journey, you should choose not to consume alcohol. I don't mean that you should cut back, or limit yourself to one glass of wine at dinner—I mean you must avoid all alcohol. Though alcohol is a spirit and can be used in ceremonies to tap into the spirit (which is why it's called spirits), it has no place in this healing protocol. For a healthy person, I think moderate and occasional alcohol consumption is fine. But as you are detoxing your body on your healing path, alcohol cannot be consumed.

Your liver plays a humongous role in detoxing your body. In fact, your liver detoxes most of the liquid content in your body—which is your blood.

Detoxification is the removal of toxins, or poisons, in the body. If your liver is not functioning optimally, your body will not be able to heal itself. Once alcohol enters your system, it impairs your liver's ability to function properly—in essence, you cannot detox the body when you have any alcohol in your system because alcohol prevents your central detoxing organ from working.

Your goal here is to achieve optimal functioning of your immune system. Drinking alcohol creates the opposite of what you are trying to accomplish!

In this phase of healing, you only want to consume foods and liquids that boost your immune system. Anything that goes against that is not allowed in your temple!

I've always been fascinated with the human body. Our body is a miracle. It's an amazing machine that heals itself all day long. However, our body needs the right ingredients to do its job. It needs the right ingredients to heal, too.

You've heard the expression garbage in, garbage out. Well, the body is the perfect example of a machine. If you put good things into the machine, you get good things out of it, like health, happiness, strength, and a good life. The reverse is also true, though. If you gunk your body up with garbage and things that are bad for it (like cigarettes, drugs, alcohol, chemicals, and empty calories), the result will be health problems, injury, stress, pain, fatigue, and even depression or anxiety.

You are what you eat is most certainly one of the truest clichés known to woman.

There are three essential, basic points that are crucial to any physical detox, once we've eliminated smoking, alcohol, and other toxins:

• Drinking good clean water and lots of it

• Eating organic, unprocessed foods

 • Taking herbs and supplements that boost your immune system

It's simple. Eliminate the bad stuff and replace it with the good stuff. If it comes from the Earth, there's a very good chance it's good for you. If it comes from a box, it's probably lost a lot of those qualities that make it so amazingly healing.

Eating whole and clean is the way to go. This does not mean you have to compromise taste. Trust me, I'm a huge foodie and I love to eat. Enjoying food is a big part of my life and eating whole and clean foods makes it all even better. The food tastes so much better when it's fresh and in it's purest form.

Water

Let's talk about water. There are some very powerful reasons to drink lots of water every day, and it's important to form this habit.

The thing about it is, we don't often focus on this habit. Instead, we drink coffee, lots of soda, and alcohol, not to mention fruit juices and milk and a bunch of other possibilities. Or just as often, we don't drink enough fluids. Drinking at least 8 glasses of water is essential for good health, especially when you're detoxing your body.

I recommend drinking 10 to 12 glasses of water daily while you are on the healing protocol. It's important to start your day with a glass of warm (not cold) water, so the first thing that enters your body upon waking is warm water, which aids your body in producing the first bowel movement. I like to sip on hot tea throughout the day; I enjoy the soothing sensation of drinking warm water.

BMs

I love talking about bowel movements and digestion, because it's a very important topic. When you are healing your body naturally with foods and supplements, you must, must, *must* take care of your digestive system—not before, not after, but while you are doing everything else. A healthy digestive system allows your body to actually absorb the healing properties from the foods. Without it, the healing benefits of the foods are not effectively absorbed.

There are three important elements for a healthy digestive system:

• Warm water and relaxation every morning when you wake up. Take the time to wake up in the morning, do your meditation, and drink warm water. Give yourself some time to have your first BM. I like to boil ginger in water and drink it with green tea.

• Probiotics. Healthy bacteria are super important for a healthy digestive system and they help to produce big, healthy bowel movements.

• Fiber-filled smoothies. We'll get more into that in the next chapter. For now, remember these smoothies are one corner of the healthy digestive system triangle.

Keeping a glass bottle or BPA free plastic bottle on you and filling it with fresh water throughout the day makes drinking water easy. Fruit juice, or any other juice, is not a replacement for water. Water is water, but not all water is the same. I don't recommend drinking tap water— most tap water is filled with trash, chemicals, and fluoride, all of which you want to keep out of your body during your healing journey.

Reverse Osmosis water is the best water, in my opinion. It's clean and stripped of all of the chemicals and trash that may come in tap water. Most health food stores have reverse osmosis water you can fill up yourself in big gallon jugs. That's probably your best bet.

I also want to mention alkaline water and alkaline water machines. This is not necessary for your healing – but it's great if you have one and can drink alkaline water. Our bodies are made up of 75% water—and for most people, that water is more acidic than alkaline, which makes the body vulnerable to viruses and infection. Viruses cannot and will not survive in an alkaline environment.

Coffee

This brings me to the topic of coffee. Coffee is extremely acidic, which is the reason it is banned from the healing protocol. Under "normal" circumstances, a little coffee, in moderation, is fine. But like cigarettes and alcohol, coffee has too great of a negative impact—in fact, it can reverse the results you are seeking to achieve. So when detoxing, coffee is forbidden.

A good replacement for coffee is Yerba Mate. Yerba Mate (yer-bah mah■tay) is made from the naturally caffeinated and nourishing leaves of a holly tree in the rainforest.

Benefits of Yerba Mate include:

• Helps stimulate focus and clarity

• Boosts physical energy

• Aids elimination

• Contains antioxidants

Eating Organic and Non-Processed Foods

When I learned I had HPV and decided to heal myself, I took a good look at everything I was eating. Though I was eating healthy, when I really looked at the labels on my groceries, I found that many of them were not organic and packed with chemicals. I knew I had to clean up the foods I ate.

Before I got HPV, I didn't value organic foods and thought buying them was a big waste of money. What's the big deal, anyway?? Well, first, it's an illusion that organic foods seem more expensive. Government subsidies for high-tech, chemical-laden farming causes non-organic foods to have lower prices. However, if we add the health and environmental costs to such products, they are ultimately far more expensive. The long-term cost of eating non-organic vs. organic — with health costs, medical costs, etc., far exceeds the cost of eating organic.

As 11-year-old Birke Baehr said, "You're either gonna pay the farmers or you're gonna pay the hospitals". (if you have not seen Birke's remarkable talk, check him out Ted.com)

The human body can only function, and do so properly, when it is well, or rather, healthy. The body stays in good health when it receives organic foods necessary to maintain vitality, and these nutrients come from the food we eat.

Some of the "healthiest foods," i.e., the foods highest in essential nutrients and for our purposes that are also familiar, affordable, and great tasting, are the same foods that are artificially, chemically, synthetically, and genetically produced. As a result, when we consume these foods, the human body is not only being robbed of the nutrients it needs to sustain itself, but it is also being exposed to dangerous chemicals that can cause serious harm.

It's a no-brainer that we must eat organic foods as part of a healthy, healing lifestyle.

What are organic foods?

Organic food is food that is derived from plants and animals that is produced without the use of synthetic fertilizers, artificial pesticides, herbicides, antibiotics, growth hormones, feed additives, or genetically modified organisms (GMOs).

Natural does not constitute organic. Natural is a

term that many grocers and consumers use to describe foods that have been minimally processed or contain no preservatives. Natural foods may include organic foods, but not all natural foods are organic.

There is also a huge amount of "organic junk food" out in the market, like organic cookies and other processed goods. These are okay occasionally but should not be consumed regularly.

Also, it's very important to note that there are some foods that are much more heavily sprayed than others, and these are the one you should never, EVER eat non- organic.

The following chart show the most pesticide contaminated earth foods. Imagine someone holding up a can of Raid and spraying it on to your beautiful raspberries. Um... GROSS!

- Apples
- Bell peppers
- Celery
- Cherries
- Grapes *(imported)*
- Nectarines
- Peaches
- Pears
- Potatoes
- Red Raspberries
- Spinach
- Strawberries

From www.organic.org

Switching to non-processed food means you will be making most of your meals yourself. That means that you won't be purchasing or eating most prepared, frozen, canned, or pre-cooked. You'll be cooking from scratch, using the best foods available in their most natural unaltered state.

There is something so powerful and divine about preparing your own healing meals. You are at the SOURCE of what goes into your body—from buying it to making it, it's all in your hands. You have the key to heal yourself, and you are using it. Yay!

Healing Foods Grocery List:

Avocado: One avocado a day, that's the staple. Avocadoes are an AMAZING healing food. They are the second highest food in glutathione, a super-duper important phytochemical that activates phase II detoxification of your liver. Remember, boosting your liver's functions is vital to your healing. It's a huge part of your detoxification program. So saying yes to avocado and no to alcohol makes your liver super happy and helps it to work super hard for you and your healing.

Beets: Beets beat the disease! I include half a

beet everyday in my smoothie. You can also chop them up and eat them in a salad. The healing properties of beets are maximized when beets are eaten raw, so don't cook them. Beets are AMAZING and super efficient at cleaning your blood, which is the main source of liquid in your body, where viruses and bacteria live. Beets will zap out that unhealthy stuff and leave your blood healthy and bright.

Garlic: Garlic is earth's gift to us in the form of a powerful antibiotic, anti-virus, anti-bacteria food! It's phenomenal stuff! I keep a cilantro-garlic pesto in my fridge at all times, and I swear by it! It's a part of my daily diet and it keeps me healthy. I don't get colds, the flu, or any other seasonal illnesses. Trust me, garlic is your friend.

Apples: One Apple A Day keeps the Doc Away. Period. Make sure they are organic.

Asparagus: I consider asparagus a super food. Asparagus has the most glutathione content of any food on the planet! It's a super duper cleanser and helps to detox the liver—therefore, asparagus is a *must eat* every day! I boil a little asparagus every day and put it in a Tupperware container to snack on throughout the day. Make sure you drink lots of water—especially when eating asparagus—as you are cleansing the body and it needs to be flushed out with tons of water. So drink up!

Coconut: There are two foods that are known to kill viruses: raw garlic and coconut. Coconut is a super-food that is a must in this healing protocol. Use coconut oil to cook with and eat lots of coconut meat. Snack on dried coconut flakes and throw them in your smoothies.

Kale: Kale is a very rich source of greens. It is a superstar in the arena of antioxidants and also aids in digestion! It packs a bunch of vitamin K, which is one of those really important vitamins we all need to get.

Aloe Vera: Aloe Vera has magical healing properties- and for healing HPV this gift from Earth's soil is ESSENTIAL. The best way to take Aloe Vera is in your smoothie in the morning. Buy the whole leaf or grow your own plant. Do not eat the outer skin, scoop out the jelly inside.

Kiwi: Vitamin C madness. Put it whole in your smoothies.

Ginger: For your morning tea, this will help your digestion and leave you feeling groovy.

The magic ingredient:

Beta-Mannan

Yes, this is the magic ingredient to this healing formula, at least in the food healing chapter. Everything else in this chapter can and will keep anyone super healthy and feeling great, but the Beta-Mannan is specific to the condition of HPV.

Dr. Joe Glickman from the website www.alotek.com created an all natural Aloe Vera-based supplement called Beta-Mannan, which has safely eliminated HPV-related illnesses in 90 days or less in the vast majority of cases for thousands of men and women who have followed the treatment recommendations with Beta-Mannan, including myself.

Its ingredients are a nutritional food supplement, and it contains a very specific combination of extracts and concentrates of the healing compounds found in Aloe Vera. It is completely natural and organic. You can take the capsules both orally and vaginally.

Let's take a breath together here…

I am certain that my healing was a combination of the spiritual, mental, and physical work I did and improvements I made. I am also clear that this supplement played a vital part in me being HPV-free. It's the key element for healing HPV- but it's important to understand that all the other elements must be in place for this to work. You must clean out your system, boost your immune system, exercise, and be at peace. You must also be positive to allow healing energy to do its work, and meditate so these elements can work together in order to have a healthy lifestyle and healthy mind. Then, you can really create the ultimate space for healing your body of HPV.

Exercise:

What do you eat right now that is healing your body? What are you eating right now that is impairing the healing?

11 LOVE YOURSELF
(AND MEAN IT!)

My motto is "Love your self and all will come." The more I preach this, the more I see how much work I have to do on myself in this area! I guess that's why they say, "You teach what you need to learn the most," huh?

I remember looking at myself in the mirror one morning, not long after I found out I had HPV, and noticing the negative familiar thoughts racing through my mind.

"You're *such a loser.*" "*You're not good enough.*"

"*You don't deserve any of these good things.*" And I said: "STOP! *Enough is Enough!!!*" I kept talking to myself as I looked in the mirror:

"Zee, *you've being nasty to yourself for way too long now. It's just gotten old, you know, sweetie? You just can't run this show anymore. Enough is enough. Time to let it go.*"

"*I will NOT, I repeat, **I will not** tolerate this behavior anymore. I will not listen to that* *bulls$%*% anymore."*

"Zee, it's time. It's time to really, really love yourself and MEAN IT!"

That was a pivotal moment for me. All the self-love rituals, mantras, and yoga had led me to this. One moment became a remarkable shift. In that moment, I knew I couldn't go on like this anymore. I was on a healing journey, and healing's #1 ingredient is love—deep, juicy, generous, full, sweet, yummy, real and authentic, unconditional LOVE.

I finally got it. If I didn't believe I was worthy, I wasn't going to treat myself or my body as if I was. Think about it. If you don't care about an animal or a plant, you're probably not going to be attentive to it or nurture and care for it as much as you would if you really, really loved it.

Unconditional love is the strongest part of our desire, willingness, and ability to overcome anything. And I had to give it to myself. No amount of love from anyone else would equal or have the same effect as the love I could offer myself.

Before HPV, I didn't have a "strong" enough reason to "really love myself and mean it." I did my best to be good to myself, do the things I knew encouraged self-love, but it was all inauthentic.

You could say that I took myself for granted. What happens when you take another person for granted? They feel unappreciated, unimportant, and they begin to move away from us. Finally, I began to really appreciate myself. This time, I knew I was tapping into the real thing.

I took another look in the mirror.

"It's okay, ZeeZee. I love you, girl, and we're gonna do this together. You are so freaking beautiful, a shining star, and I love you. I love you. I love you. And you are perfect just the way you are, HPV and all. (laugh). Yes, HPV, anal warts and all, girl. You are perfect."

The floodgates of tears opened up, and I let it out—all of the ugly self-defeating poisons that had dwelled within me for years. I released all the shame, the guilt, the disgust, the resentment, and all of the anger (especially the anger that was self-directed)... it all came out in my tears and my sobs, my entire body was crying. Believe me, it was a powerful cleansing and release.

The pain and the hurt I had caused myself had marked me, year after year, thought after thought. I had hit the wall, the turning point, and there was no going back to the old way. I was done with it, and I was relieved—a little scared, but relieved. Because now I was starting fresh—from a place of real love—it was a place I liked, but not a place I knew very well.

My fear stemmed from being afraid of the unknown. If I stopped bad-mouthing myself in my head, what would I do now? That's the only thing I knew. Now, I was left with a big blank space. It felt awkwardly uncomfortable, but I also knew that what was comfortable was unacceptable. So I sat in this new space for a while, scared and exhilarated. This was new beginning for me, and I needed to take some time to get to know this new perspective, this new way of thinking.

Loving yourself means so many different things to different people. What does it mean to you? Does it mean that you accept your limitations? Or does it mean that you stop beating yourself up, learning to love your imperfections, your body, your mind, your capacity to learn, grow, love and live? Regardless of what it means to you, learning how to love yourself starts with a conscious decision to love yourself *unconditionally*. That means you accept the good and the bad, including your HPV and everything that comes with it. You can't love part of yourself, while wishing you could change another part. You're a whole package, and every part of your being is what makes you who you are.

Women, especially, often criticize and judge themselves far too harshly. We don't give ourselves credit where credit is due. We make far too many unreasonable expectations on ourselves which, by the way, sets us up to fail. Learning to truly love yourself is a healing journey on its own, so give yourself time. It requires a conscious awareness of your self- beliefs and judgments. As you become more and more aware of the destructive conversations you have in your head about yourself, it may feel like you are not getting anywhere, but remember awareness and acceptance are the first two steps toward healing. Once you've made them, you're well on your way.

1. Stop All Criticism. Criticism never changes a thing. You can put yourself down until you're blue in the face, and guess what? Whatever it is that sparked your disapproval will still be there when you're done. Refuse to criticize yourself. Accept yourself exactly as you are.

This is especially true when you criticize yourself for your current situation.

How did you react when you found out you had HPV? Did you judge yourself? Go back to the exercise we did in Chapter 3. What was your answer to the question "What does the fact that you "got" HPV mean about you?" This is your opportunity to change that answer, because, truthfully, the fact that you have HPV means nothing about you. You are still the person that you are, but now you are a person who has a virus. Nothing about that changes the unique magnificence that is you, and only you.

2. Forgive Yourself. Let go of the past. Dwelling on what is done and over only allows it to live on—it gives the past too much power and control over today and tomorrow. We all make mistakes. We're human. We don't come equipped with all the right answers. That's what life is about—living and learning. Mistakes are nothing more than learning activities. Let the past go! You did the best you could at the time with the understanding, awareness, and knowledge that you had. Now you are growing and changing, and you will live life differently. For that reason, your past is your friend—it has made you a better person. It's taught you lessons that make you smarter, wiser, and less likely to do or say anything in the future that you might regret.

Tell yourself: "I forgive you for the things you did in the past that did not serve you. I know you did the best you can do in every moment. I forgive you and I love you."

These are powerful words to utter to yourself. They are some of the greatest healing words in the world.

3. Don't Scare Yourself. Stop terrorizing yourself with your thoughts. Thinking about the, "what ifs," can be a very dangerous place to go. What if this doesn't work? What if I get cancer? What if I can't have kids?

It's true that most of the things we worry about don't happen. Worrying is a waste of time. It creates fear based on possibilities, not probabilities. Stay in the present, focus on the positive and be here now. "What if?" should never be a question. It means you're trying to deal with something that doesn't yet exist. Why waste your time and energy on something that isn't, when you can focus on today, right now, and what really is?

4. Be Gentle and Kind and Patient. Be gentle with yourself. Be kind to yourself. Be patient with yourself as you learn new ways of thinking. Treat yourself as you would treat someone you really loved—physically and emotionally, with words and with actions.

Too often, we give strangers more courtesy and kindness than we give to ourselves. You wouldn't walk up to a stranger and say, "Hey, fatso, you're a disgrace. Here, have this candy bar. It'll make your waistline grow and make you feel sluggish. When you're done eating it, I want you to beat yourself up and hate yourself for it." You wouldn't dream of doing that to a stranger, but how often do you do that to yourself? How often do you treat your body poorly, then turn around and hate yourself? When was the last time that you did something kind for your body and your self-esteem? When was the last time that you treated yourself with the compassion, kindness, and respect that you give to others?

I could write an entire book on being kind and patient with ourselves, and someday, I might. For now, though, know that you cannot attain a healthy body or mind until you are able to be patient with yourself—healing takes time, nurturing takes time, transformation, change, and new habits take time. Be kind and give yourself that time. Only then will you be able to enjoy the results it brings.

5. Be Kind to Your Mind. Self-hatred is nothing more than the hatred of your own thoughts. Don't hate yourself for having those thoughts.

Observe them as they come and go and know that you, the real you, is not your thoughts. You are so much more than your thoughts, girl! Plus, most of your thoughts are totally not true and a little wacky, right? Maybe you can laugh about it once in a while! Also, be aware that because you are not your thoughts, you can change your thoughts at any time! Now that's a powerful tool that you can use to enhance your life and your health, and it is available to you all day, every day!

6. Praise Yourself. Tell yourself how well you are doing with every little thing. At the end of each day, make a list of the 10 things you accomplished today. It doesn't matter if they are large or small. An accomplishment is something to celebrate. Pat yourself on the back! Give yourself a "job well done." This is an amazingly effective exercise and will get you present to all the amazing things you do that you forget to praise yourself for.

Today, I praise myself for:

Eating healthy foods.

Having positive thoughts.

Enjoying the sunrise.

Reaching out to a friend.

Being kind to myself.

7. Support Yourself. Find ways to support yourself. Reach out to friends and allow them to help you. You are being strong when you ask for help when you need it. Share this book with your close friends and let them know what you're creating— you're creating a healthier body, a healthier lifestyle, and a fantastic, nurturing, caring mindset that will support it. You will be surprised at the response you get and the support that will show up for you. Plus, it will allow other women to open up to you, and you may find that more women than you imagined are affected by HPV—and would love to know what you are learning!

8. Take Care of Your Body. Begin to follow the food healing protocols covered in the Appendix. Put those healing foods in your body.

Take warm Epsom salt baths at least once a week (stay in the bath for 20 minutes at least and allow yourself to absorb the healing energy of the salts). Practice yoga, go hiking, walking, swimming, and dancing. Your body is your spaceship in this life—enjoy it and treat it well.

9. Do Mirror Work. Look into your eyes often. Express the growing sense of love you have for yourself. Forgive yourself while looking in the mirror. Talk to your parents while looking into the mirror. Forgive them, too. Forgive your former partners, your spouse, your sister, your boss. Cleanse yourself of the past and fill yourself with approval, acceptance, and love. At least once a day, say, "I love you, I really love you!"

10. Have Fun. Remember the things that gave you joy as a child and do them now. Find a way to have fun with everything you do. Make fun the ingredient that turns your life into a fantastic adventure!

11. Forgive yourself and others. Forgiveness is a crucial element in healing. When we hold on to resentment, anger, and contempt, it only hurts us. Being angry about anything is destructive to our body and our spirit.

Harboring anger, resentment, or negative feelings about an experience or a person only hurts us. It's also true that holding onto the anger, the hurt, and the pain is self-sabotaging. It's like a poison that infiltrates into everything we do and prevents us from living a life of peace and happiness.

We cannot possibly reach our full potential, our optimal health, and true joy if we carry resentment, anger, or contempt throughout our lives. Forgiving those who we feel have wronged or hurt us or others will free our hearts, minds, and souls from the self-imposed barriers that anger builds around us. It's like a huge burden being lifted from our mind and heart, allowing us to sigh in relief and move on in our lives!

Our time is limited—let's not waste one more day feeling angry about the past. We have no power to change what has happened, but we can change our reaction to it. We can keep it from creating more damage by letting it go, forgiving, and moving on. Put the past behind you and don't give it the power to destroy your future. Forgive and let live.

Exercise:

Who in your life have you not forgiven? Who are you withholding your love from? Who do you feel resentment toward?

Write this person a letter telling them how you feel, how they hurt you and the impact their actions or words have had on your life. Then, tell them you forgive them. Say it out loud. Feel it in your heart.

You don't ever have to read this letter to anyone other than yourself. Simply writing this and declaring that you forgive this person will release the hurt in your heart.

Remember forgiveness is an act of love... self-love.

12 FIND BIGGER PROBLEMS THAN YOURS (AND BE OF SERVICE)

If you think you have problems, look around you. NO really, look around you. Turn on the news. Read the newspaper. Surf the Internet. When you take the focus off of YOU, you will see people with bigger, more serious problems than you.

When we are faced with a challenging problem, we tend to be super egocentric, meaning we think life revolves around us and around our BIG problem. But in reality, life goes on, people keep doing what they are doing, and in the big picture, our problems aren't as monumental as we perceive them to be.

Here's an example. Lilly is consumed with the problems in her life. Her credit card bills are astronomical, and creditors are calling all the time. Her car is making funny noises, and she is worried it is going to break down and she won't have the money to fix it. Her best friend has a new boyfriend and won't return her calls anymore. The convenience store is no longer carrying her favorite organic moisturizer, and her skin is becoming very dry. Lilly is constantly thinking and talking about her problems. She identifies herself as her problems.

In Lily's head, Lilly = her problems.

Late one night, Lilly was walking from the coffee shop and was hit by a car while crossing the street. She ended up in the emergency room that night, finding herself surrounded by her family. Her best friend was there, too. Thankfully, Lilly was only slightly injured and she's going to be okay. As Lilly opened her eyes and looked at her family and friends, she realized that all the little things she was obsessively worrying about really didn't matter. In that moment, all her little problems had disappeared. This is quite amazing, because a few hours before, they seemed so real, so tangible, so in her face! And now, it's as if they were completely erased, eradicated... as if they didn't exist.

But nothing changed. Those "problems" are still there, nothing had changed "out there." What has changed is that Lilly saw a bigger problem – possibly losing her life! – and this gave the perception or the appearance that the other problems had disappeared.

Many people have similar experiences. Something BIG, critical, or life-threatening happens, something big enough for them to wake up and realize what is really important. They need a big bad hairy problem to show up so they can realize that all their other problems are small, meaningless, or even really minuscule!!

Here's the good news...you don't have to wait for a big, scary, life-threatening problem to come into your life and make your little problem seem small. You can create a big enough problem by yourself. Look around you! What's a big huge problem that is worthwhile of your attention, even worthwhile of your life? What inspires you? Where do you want to make a difference? In contrast to that problem, your own problems diminish and become less mounting, less threatening.

A few years ago, I was being sued for millions of dollars. This was scary as heck for me. It consumed my entire life. I had nightmares about people chasing me and people killing me. I was depressed and wanted to sleep most of the time.

I identified myself as this huge problem. Me = my problems. When I talked to people, I introduced myself as my problem. I made sure they knew about my problems—it would not be complete without them knowing about my problems. It felt incomplete not to tell people about my problems—because my problems were who I was. So if you knew me, you had to know my problems. We were one and the same, inseparable.

So I decided to find a problem worthy of my life and my energy. Life is full of problems, nothing is perfect or as we want it to be. We can make a difference in our community, which in turns makes a difference with the entire planet.

We just love to talk about our problems. I did. But I knew that I'd given that problem too much power and control over my life and my health. So I decided to find or create a bigger problem than my big problem. I asked myself, "What am I passionate about? Where did I want to put my energy?" The answer: I want to work with young women, teach them yoga, empower them to know who they really are and really trust in themselves."

There are millions and billions of young women on the planet that I can reach out to, one by one. So I began where I was. I started filming videos on my YouTube station. I reached out to the young women I knew and got them involved in my life and projects. Every moment in my life and everyone I met became an opportunity for me to get out of my problems and move into something bigger than myself.

Once you begin to focus on bigger problems than your own, your problems start to appear really small, and they will disappear.

Being of service does not mean we are less than or subservient to anyone or anything. It's a way of being that invites grace and abundance in our daily lives. Being of service means giving to others without expecting anything back.

It's really that simple, and the bottom-line result of such simple kindnesses is a far-reaching self-esteem, a love for yourself. Therein lies the key of self-healing: Absolute love and forgiveness for one's self.

By being of service to others, for no other reason than to be of service, you increase your love and appreciation for yourself, which results in allowing yourself to have what you want in life and letting go of what you don't want and don't need.

The beauty of it is, by leading by example, you will be helping others love and appreciate themselves and have what they want, too. That's win/win.

Exercise:

Make a list of things you are passionate about. Where do you know you can make a difference? What hardship have you overcome in your life? How can you help others who have gone through the same thing? What wisdom does your experience have to offer?

FINAL NOTE FROM THE AUTHOR

Alright, here's the deal: there is no quick fix. I made this book as short as I could so you could get through this information and get on with your beautiful life.

I wanted to share a few more tidbits in this last portion of the book of things I wanted to touch upon. Most of what's in this chapter was added after I re-read the manuscript and made notes of all the things I had missed.

Should I do surgery?

One thing I want to make clear is I am not a medical doctor and I am not giving professional advice. I am an intuitive healer (I did not know I had this gift until I got HPV and reversed it).

Listen to what your doctor tells you and listen to your heart and use your best judgment on how to proceed. If they recommend surgery, it's fine to do it if you feel good about it. The surgery will get rid of the symptoms- and that is great.

It's important to sit in your meditation and listen for your hearts higher purpose.

In fact, this book can be applicable to minor to major health issues, just swap out the word HPV for another dis-ease and read it from that perspective.

Should I tell all my ex-boyfriends?

I feel the only person who can really answer this question is you. Only you know who it is necessary to share with.

I do feel that during the healing process, who you share with is very important.

Tune in and really ask yourself- who do I want to share this with? Who do I know will support me in this process?

I was terrified to inform my ex-partners but I did and it felt good to share with them. I have really great relationships with all me "exes", so it felt "right" for me.

Can I keep having sex with my partner?

Please remember that this is all my opinion. You have to meditate on this question and feel in your heart what feels the best to you.

Personally, I felt I needed to heal my relationship with my vagina and the areas surrounding it and refraining from sexual intercourse made sense to me.

My symptoms appeared as warts- and they freaked me out at first. I wondered if I'd ever be "into" sex again. Having warts on your body does not feel good anywhere- especially not on your sexual parts. It's does not feel very sexy.

Your sexual confidence may take a plummet for a moment- but know that this too shall pass.

You've been given an opportunity to heal your relationship with your body and your sexuality.

Get this: you healing yourself and being powerful through all of this is sexy as heck. Your sexiness is no longer defined by popular culture. You are a goddess dealing with human things and your beauty and your sexiness go beyond warts, beyond wrinkles, beyond love handles. You are beautiful, period.

Conclusion

Enjoy the ride. You are a beautiful, amazing human being and you can do this. Trust me, if I'm able to do it, so can you.

If you fall off the wagon, eat the wrong things or have an emotional breakdown, chill out! Don't beat yourself up. Remember guilt is unhealthy for the mind and body. Guilt, can be as damaging, if not worse, than any chemicals you may ingest! And don't feel guilty about feeling guilty either. Listen, every day the sun rises is an opportunity to keep riding that wagon.

This is a lifelong journey! This is the only body you've got so taking care of it is an every day, 24 hour, minute-to-minute job you've got. It never stops and you can't take a break from it.

We must keep educating ourselves, listening to our own bodies and making the necessary adjustments in our lifestyle, habits and our thoughts.

If you've read this far, then you're ready to be in action in your life and making those changes you know you need to make to live a healthier, happier life.

For ongoing support and education, visit www.thankyouforhpv.com , a website created especially for you, to support you on your journey.

I acknowledge you for reading this book, for waking up this morning, for being awesome, for doing all those things you do to better yourself and the world. I acknowledge you for being willing to make a commitment for yourself, for your well being, for the world.

I look forward to hearing from you at

www.thankyouforhpv.com

HEALING RECIPES

Key Lime Pie

This pie is a staple in my kitchen. I keep one in the freezer at all times, and I have it almost every day. Avocadoes are an amazing food. Of course, they supply us with healthy fats in healthy quantities—but they also contain a great amount glutathione (#2 after asparagus), which helps the detoxing of the liver. Limes are amazing also and have anti-cancer properties. Coconut oil is a super food and is anti-bacterial and anti-viral, making it very important to eat in your healing protocol. The almonds in the crust are important in oxygenating the blood.

Crust:

2 cups almonds
3/4 cups dates (soaked in water for 10 minutes)
1/8 cup water

Blend ingredients and coat pie pan with crust

Filling:

4 large hass avocados
Juice of 10 limes
1 cup coconut oil
3 cups agave nectar

Blend the above ingredients and fill pie pan above the crust

Freeze pie. To serve, take out and allow to thaw for 30 minutes.

Creamy Garlic-Cilantro Pesto

This is a must! Make a batch and keep it in the fridge. A nice glass container to store this in is ideal. I usually make a double batch. This is a delicious medicinal spread I recommend having every day. The creamy part comes from the cashews. Adding a little extra olive oil also gives it a nice feel if you like that kind of thing. I love starting my day with it and topping it off with half of a ripe avocado.

Garlic is a natural anti-bacterial, antibiotic, anti-aging, anti-DISEASE food! It's mother earth's gift to us: it promotes optimal health and the prevention of disease. As long as I am getting tons of raw garlic in my system daily and consistently, I know I am being proactive in warding off unnecessary illness, colds, viruses, etc.

Cilantro is known to be one of the top chelators of heavy metals in the body. We all have various stages of heavy metal poisoning in our bodies, and it impacts our performance, as well as how we feel in everyday life.

Ingredients:

One head of garlic

One bunch of cilantro
One cup of olive oil
One cup of cashews

Blend and refrigerate.

Asparagus a la Asian el dente

Asparagus should be eaten every day. It's the best natural source of glutathione (glutathione= happy liver= healthy blood and body)

Ingredients:

Asparagus
Nama Shoyu (or soy sauce)
Sesame Seeds

Steam asparagus for 5 to 8 minutes only—do not overcook. They should be slightly crunchy.

Drizzle with Nama Shoyu, sesame seeds and serve.

Grapefruit Slushie

Grapefruits should be eaten daily. They have amazing healing properties and are an anti-cancer food. It's important to peel as little of the white fuzz around and inside the grapefruit; the fuzz is where the healing phytochemicals are contained.

Ingredients:

2 grapefruits
Ice

Peel and half each grapefruit. Don't remove the white fuzz around or inside the grapefruit- this is where the medicine is! Blend with ice, and serve immediately.

Macca Pudding

Macca is powerful adaptogen, which means that it boosts the body's ability to adapt to external conditions aka stress. As an adaptogen, macca works broadly to contribute to overall well being. It nourishes and calms yo' nerves and it's also really important in helping your endocrine system- which basically regulates all your hormones. As a woman, it's super duper crucial that you consume it. It's super she-hero food. For the men too, it increases sperm count for men by a gazillion (just kidding, don't quote me on that one). It's like the yoga of foods. It's a must for any and all women.

In this recipe, we mix macca with Manuka honey, a very healing honey. It can be found at health food stores. Any raw honey will work also.

Ingredients:

2 tablespoons of macca
2 tablespoons of cocoa powder
 1 cup /manuka honey
1/4 cup warm water

Mix and serve. Can be refrigerated.

Ginger Tea with Gogi Berries

This is perfect for your morning drink—it should be the first thing to enter your system upon waking in the morning. Ginger has amazing properties. It is an anti-inflammatory so it helps to manage chronic pain in the body. Goji berries have a ridiculous amount of quality vitamin C. Yum. You can also add Agave if you like it sweet. I do.

Ingredients:

1⁄2 gallon of water with 2 hands full of goji berries
 2 inch piece of ginger, chopped

Boil for 30-60 minutes and serve. You can also refrigerate to make iced ginger tea.

Healing Smoothie

This smoothie is hardcore. Hardcore healing ,
that is. Everything that goes into this smoothie is
a magical food that will make your body squeal
from the inside out. Your cells and your heart
and your liver and your stomach and your
colons- they'll all thank you. And so will your
skin, and your hair and your nails!

Ingredients:

1/4 - 1/2 organic cucumber
1/4 to 1/2 organic beet
1-2 whole organic apple
avocado with the seed (do not include the skin
and include seed only if using 3HP Vitamix or
Blendtec)
1 organic celery stalk
1/2 organic lime (peel green parts, keep white)
piece of organic ginger
fresh aloe vera (do not include skin)
add filtered water or coconut water

Blend all above ingredient and drink
immediately.

Shentrition Sunshine Juice

Shentrition is not just another green powder. It is an amazing mix of super foods. The base is hempseeds with an amazing mix of adaptogens and greens. I love to mix it with fresh squeezed orange juice. It tastes really good and it will make you feel a million times better physically and mentally. You can buy it at www.shentrition.com

Ingredients:

1 spoon Shentrition
1 cup orange juice

ABOUT THE AUTHOR

Zayna De Gaia, teacher and student, leads workshops and classes worldwide on health, nutrition, meditation and yoga. She also leads Women Healing Circles. She blogs and vlogs on her website , www.zeeluv.com, chants and sings and plays the harmonium in a kirtan band for the bliss of it and makes a mean raw vegan chocolate cupcake. She's a nomadic gypsy and lives on earth with her man and her dog. She can be found under a tree. This is her first book.

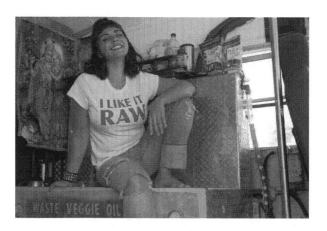

Made in the USA
Lexington, KY
30 September 2015